DEDICATION

To my parents, Carmel and Ivy who never stop believing in me.

PRAISE FROM OTHER PEOPLE ABOUT THIS BOOK

"If Only Hair Could Talk" by Lorna Jones is built upon the idea that your hair is alive and talk to you about how it is feeling.

Clearly, I can see as a hair scientist that this is not actually the case, but it is a really nice way of communicating to people how, sometimes, they need to be more considerate of their hair. How they need to adapt their diet and lifestyle to help it grow as healthily as possible, and how they need to always try to minimise hair damage.

The book gives some essential tips that will help consumers become better friends with their own hair.

Dr Paul Cornwell
TRI Princeton

CONTENTS

ACKNOWLEDGEMENTS

Thank you, David Salinger Certified Trichologist and Course Director, International Association of Trichologists (IAT) in Sydney, Australia. David provided me with the learning opportunity to undertake my trichology education. He has been a constant source of inspiration and support without which none of this would have been possible.

Thank you, Evie Johnson Certified Trichologist and member of the Board of Directors (IAT) in Maryland, United States of America. Evie provided me with hope, when all was lost during a period when my hair refused to stay on my head. Not only did she assist in bringing my hair back to its rightful place, she also encouraged me to share my story, to inspire other people. I have not looked back.

Thank you, to all my family and friends who have joined me on this amazing journey and who never stop encouraging me.

I salute you all.

FOREWARD

I first met Lorna in 2018, at the International Association of Trichologists (IAT) conference in Washington DC. After the conference, she started studying Trichology and seeking knowledge from trichologists, from all across the globe. Her travels took her to the: United States; United Kingdom; Australia; South Africa; Holland; and to our most recent IAT Trichology conference in Canada, where Lorna lectured. Between the two conferences, she successfully completed a Trichology Course and opened two clinics. It makes me exhausted thinking about all that she has achieved in such a short time, but it provides you with an idea of the sort of person Lorna is.

The wonderful thing about hair is that however much we abuse it, new replaces damaged. How many other things do you know that are always coming back for more punishment? However, of course the less we damage our hair, the better it looks and many things we do to our hair can damage it, if not done correctly.

This book is written from the hair's point of view with the objective of encouraging you to look after your hair. Hair loss is often the first sign of an internal imbalance, when a trip to a qualified Trichologist such as Lorna, can help you on your way to pinpointing the cause. Excessive hair loss normally relates to internal imbalances, including: medical problems; nutritional deficiencies; and medications being taken etc. There are problems that correct themselves but others that require help. Your hair is not only for beauty but is also an indication of your: physical and mental health; immune problems; hormonal problems; nutritional imbalances; and stress, which all affect your hair health and condition. The more you learn about hair, the more amazing you realise it is.

Enjoy this excellent book.

David Salinger

Director, International Association of Trichologists, Australia

IF ONLY HAIR COULD TALK

PREFACE

This book is for this and our next generation

I imagined that if my hair could talk, what it would have said to me during a time when I experienced hair loss.

You see, I believe your hair generally speaks to you, quietly, and tells you what it needs and what it wants. You only have to pay attention to it, to understand what it is saying.

For the purposes of this book, I have given my hair the superpower ability to allow it to speak out loud.

While this book does not go into detailed facts about hair loss, it features 'good gentle grooming' practices, which provide useful tips for women with afro-textured hair. It is written primarily, but not exclusively, for people with, and with an interest in, afro-textured hair.

This book is designed to be educational and informative in a fun way. It will appeal to anyone eager to learn about this type of hair texture and associated hair care practices.

What do you think your hair would say to you, if only hair could talk?

CHAPTER ONE

HAIR

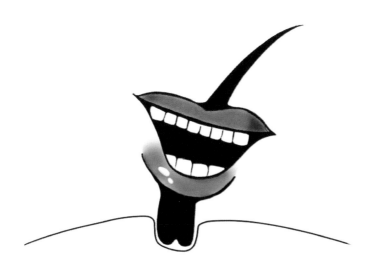

Hair grows from a root called a bulb, exactly like a plant, which is located deep in the scalp. If you cut it, it won't hurt because it is not alive and has no nerve endings.

Let me introduce myself. My name is Hair. Well, afro-textured hair really, so you can call me AT, for short.

It is unusual that I can speak to you but I figured it would be useful to break my usual silence to have a chat, so we understand each other now I am on your scalp. You see, I would like to stay around as long as I can, but I can only do that with your help.

Let me explain.

Three months ago, my journey started when I was deep in the dermis as a hair bulb. The dermis is under your skin. It was great there because I had all the food I could possibly eat in the form of nutrients. These were delivered to me by your blood vessels and I grew and grew, until I pushed my way through the epidermis close to the skin's surface. As I grew, I took in lots of protein and became keratinised. Actually, I am completely made up of keratin.

With one final push, I had made it through to your scalp and there I was, although now I was no longer a living entity. So, at what point does hair actually stop living?

This is the tricky part. Most of me remained under the surface of the skin under your scalp and continued collecting all the nutrients from the blood vessels to keep me alive. But, the tiny bit of me on your scalp was no longer alive.

Which means that if you took a pair of scissors and cut me, I wouldn't feel it because I have no nerve endings. The only thing you can do now that I am here is to condition me, keep me nice and moisturized, and style me.

That is it.

If you cut me, I won't grow any quicker because I grow from the root, which as I said, is deep in the dermis, under your skin.

The challenge for you is to keep me going for as long as you possibly can. Mostly, this depends on the conditioning and styling of the part of me, which is on your scalp. But don't forget about my bulb too, the hair root under your scalp, which also needs care.

Right, let's begin our journey together.

CHAPTER TWO

GROWTH

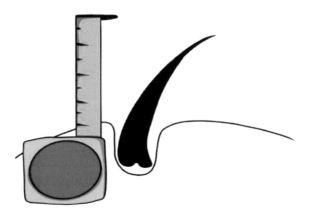

Hair grows in cycles. There are 3 distinct stages: The Anagen Stage, the growth stage, which in afro-textured hair can last between 2 to 4 years; the Catagen Stage, which lasts around a week; and the Telogen Stage, which lasts around 3 to 4 weeks.

I have been in the Anagen Stage for some time now and things have been looking good. I can stay in this Anagen, growth stage for anything between 2 to 4 years because this is the average length of turnaround time for the life of afro-textured hair. People with afro-textured hair can have short hair, medium length hair, or long hair; it depends on their genes. The longer the Anagen Stage, the longer the hair. If you have short hair, I will be around for a couple of years; if your hair is long, I will be here for around 4 years. If it is not short, but not long then I will be here on your scalp somewhere in the middle, maybe around 3 years.

At the end of the Anagen Stage, I will move into the next part of my growth cycle, which is the Catagen Stage. I will stay here for about a week; it is a holding stage, really. Nothing very much happens here. I stop growing and hang around for a week or so. After this, I will move into the Telogen Stage and this really is the end of the road for me because I am getting ready to leave you. I will fall out but that is fine because I will return!

As long as nothing has disrupted my hair growth cycle, I will be coming back in the next 3 months or so. It takes that time for me to restart the journey, from my bulb deep in the dermis, to appearing back on your scalp.

It is a continuous cycle according to the length of your hair. I work really hard to grow for up to 4 years while I am on your scalp. When I fall out, I take a 3 month break and then I come back. As mentioned earlier, as long as nothing has happened to disrupt my growth cycle, whether at the Anagen Stage or Telogen Stage, my aim is to return.

Let me tell you how you can make my 4 years on your scalp an enjoyable one.

Read on.

CHAPTER THREE

FLUIDS

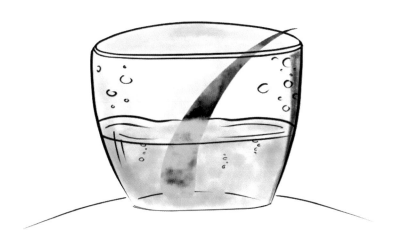

Water is necessary to sustain human life.

Hair care is self-care.

I am really thirsty. I mean, I am actually parched. Please, can you go and drink a glass of water?

You see, there are millions of cells inside your body and a fair few of those are needed to make my hair shaft and to keep me growing. These cells need water, exactly like the blood, which circulates in your body transporting all of these cells and oxygen, which also needs water.

In addition, my unique set of blood vessels, which supplies my hair bulb at the bottom of my hair shaft, really needs to be well-looked after and hydrated if I am to grow healthily.

You need water to sustain your body and I am part of your body, so please drink that glass of water, right now? Can you also ensure you have the recommended daily intake of fluids, which is around 6 to 8 glasses a day, of preferably pure natural water.

You will thank me for it later.

CHAPTER FOUR

NUTRITION

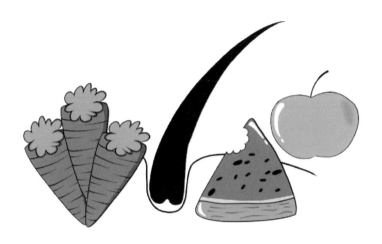

A healthy balanced diet is required to ensure you receive all the nutrients you need to sustain your vital organs and to keep your body working at its optimum.

I am feeling rather peckish. Actually, I am really hungry. Please, can you eat something, preferably something healthy?

Do you remember when I explained how I ate quite well when I was in the bulb, before I appeared on your scalp? Please don't stop now!

I can feel the blood circulating around my hair bulb, but the nutrients won't make that final leap into my blood vessels and I am starting to get a little worried.

You see, if your body is deficient in any nutrients, your brain makes an executive decision for the nutrients in your blood to bypass my hair bulb and transport them to the rest of your body first. I lose out. I know your heart, lungs, liver, kidneys and all the other vital organs in your body are important and need the nutrients the most. I get that. Well, your brain also knows you can survive without a single hair on your head and that is why I lose out…eek!

I quite like being hair and because you quite like me being here on your scalp, it is really important that you have a healthy balanced diet to ensure your body is not deficient in any nutrients. As you can see, I eat last and sometimes not at all, and this threatens my existence.

So, if it is possible, please give yourself a healthy, balanced diet, if you don't mind.

I'd like to stick around for as long as I possibly can.

CHAPTER FIVE

HEAT

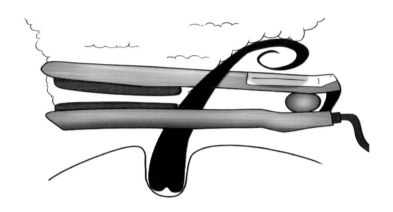

Heat straightening can cause the hair shaft to become weak. Curling tongs cause more damage than hair dryers.

Ouch! Why are you burning me with those tongs? Don't you like me? It is so hot. I am not sure if I will be able to withstand this heat. If you keep doing this to me, I may have to pack my bags and leave and I am sure you really wouldn't like that, would you?

I know you have sprayed a heat protectant product on me, which I guess is better than nothing at all, but do you really have to use so much heat to straighten me?

Considering that water boils at 100 degrees Celsius, your curling tongs are double this heat, at 230 degrees Celsius. It is way too hot for me!

You know I am naturally curly because I told you my name is AT. I know you like the straight look from time to time, but every time you use those tongs it makes me feel weak and dehydrated. This is because the bonds inside me, which hold me together become displaced and it is really uncomfortable.

If you have to use heat on me, please can you only do so occasionally, and not every week, and turn down the temperature?

The intense heat makes me feel really fragile.

CHAPTER SIX

CHEMICALS

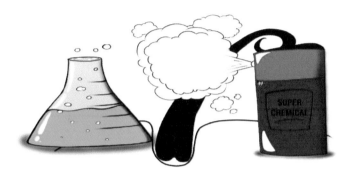

Chemical straightening removes a layer of fatty acids that is bound to the hair cuticle. This is important to prevent penetration of water into the hair shaft. Chemical straightening can cause catastrophic damage.

Aaarrgghhh! What was that you poured all over me?

I am being straightened again. Is that a chemical relaxer that you have added to me, which has turned me from curly to straight again?

I hope it is not too strong because the last time you used it, it burnt your scalp, which was really damaging. In addition, you may remember how some of my neighbours disappeared altogether. This was because certain chemicals can cause so much damage that the hair follicles die off completely and then there is no chance of any regrowth in those areas.

Also, can you please remember that I am already fragile because my hair has weak points in it every time there is a kink in my curl. Also, it is traditionally dry, again because of my curls, so when you add a chemical to me, it worries me.

Therefore, please can you take extra care of me because the chemicals will be drying. You need to ensure I am kept moisturised. I wouldn't want any part of me to get so dry that I snap off and break.

Finally, please can you ensure you do not over process me and when you re-do the process that you only put it on the regrowth, rather than all over me. This is important to make sure I don't get more damaged than I need to. Lastly, please do not relax me for at least another 2 to 3 months. Definitely, do not use those tongs on me, now that I am freshly relaxed for at least a couple of weeks. Please.

I am now in a most fragile state.

CHAPTER SEVEN

WASHDAY

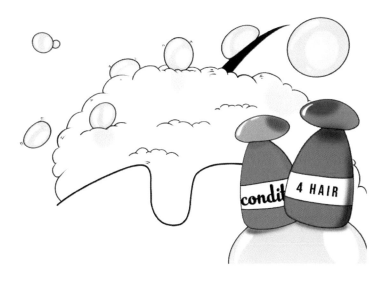

It is important to wash afro-textured hair at least weekly, to ensure you remove all the product build-up and also to maintain a clean scalp for good healthy growth.

It is washday, great! I know you don't wash me several times a week because of your need to hairstyle, but I like a good wash, at least once a week.

This is important because you spend all week putting different products on me and your scalp, so you really need to wash away all the product build-up, so I can prepare myself for some more.

Also, when you are drying me is there any chance that you could towel dry me gently, please, instead of using heat again?

I am only asking.

If you must use heat from the hair dryer, please can you have the heat on a medium level, so I am not damaged while you are drying me.

When it comes to night time and you are off to bed, please can you wrap me up in a satin or silk scarf because that is very gentle and is great for me to have a good night's rest, exactly like you.

CHAPTER EIGHT

COLOUR

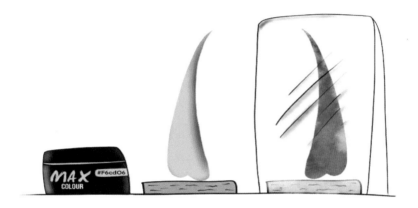

Hair is made up of 3 layers. The outer layer is called the cuticle and it protects the hair shaft. The middle layer is the cortex and the innermost layer is the medulla. Colouring hair several times a month can be damaging to the hair.

Oh, so you fancied a bit of colour, did you?

That is fine, but did you have to use those massive colour molecules? Couldn't you have used something a little less permanent?

You see, I only have 3 layers. The outer layer, the cuticle; the middle layer, the cortex; and the inside layer, the medulla.

If you had used a temporary spray-on colour, this would cover me and only affect my cuticle, my outer layer. The colour stays on usually until you wash me and this is the least intrusive process of colouring hair.

On the other hand, if you used a semi-permanent colour, this penetrates my cuticle and sits in the cortex. This lasts longer and will only wash out after about 7 or 8 washes.

If you choose to permanently colour me, this does not wash out at all. Instead it stays in my cortex. Strictly speaking, colouring hair should not cause me too many problems, but if you dye me several times a month this can be damaging and dehydrating. Also, I would rather that you didn't do it on the same day as chemically processing me.

Finally, please can you remember, if you put me out in the sun, I may fade a little. Please, can you put a nice sun hat on to keep me away from the ultra violet rays because they can be damaging, whether you have coloured me or not. Thank you.

CHAPTER NINE

WIGS

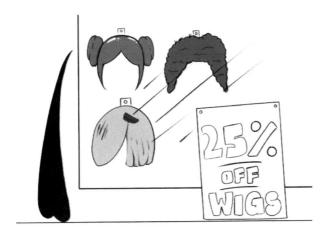

Wigs are useful to protect the hair and are great for instant transformation, but it is important also to take good care of the hair underneath.

Hey, who turned the lights out?

Okay, I get it, you are giving me a rest while you put on an instant, ready hairstyle. That is fine, as long as you don't forget about me under here.

You see, I don't mind having a little break from the constant combing and brushing, which can sometimes be too much activity for me. But you need to take care of me, too.

Let me explain.

The friction of the wig on your head can damage me, so please buy yourself a wig cap. Well, a few wig caps actually because it is so hot in here, the sweat will gather underneath the wig and on your scalp and get caught up in the wig cap. When you think about it, sweat is made up 98 per cent water and the rest is made up of other substances, including salts and urea or waste, and it needs to be washed away, frequently. Otherwise, it will end up going back into your scalp and right into my hair follicle and it doesn't feel very nice.

Therefore, a regular supply of wig caps and a regular hair washing regime is essential. Along with giving me regular opportunities to enjoy the fresh air.

Also, please do not make the wig too tight because this can cause pressure on the scalp edges and damage my hairline. This can eventually lead to you losing me around this area.

The key to good hair care, when you wear a wig, is to ensure that nothing is too tight on your head, and your scalp is regularly cleansed.

Lastly, please never consider using any glue on your scalp because when you do, you may never see me again and I am not yet ready to leave.

CHAPTER TEN

HAIRSTYLES

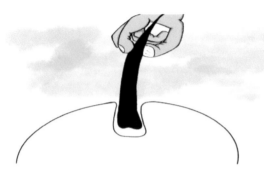

Traction Alopecia is caused by the chronic pulling of hair into a style. It leads to a thinning of the hair in that area, or loss of hair.

Some of the hairstyles you give me are my great, but I have to tell you more about them.

Locs

I loved the locs style you gave me when you decided to twist me around my pals. That was nice but it was a little bit tight and quite heavy, so the next time please, would you mind not re-twisting me so often and ensuring the twists are not too tight?

Extensions and braids

I also loved the extensions, when you added them onto me and when you braided me with the rest of my pals. The only thing I was worried about was that it was too tight. I could really do with you loosening this the next time you decide to have this hairstyle. Can you also remember, when you apply these extensions to me, I have already been chemically relaxed, so you are storing up trouble and we don't want that do we? Can you please, release me from those braids every 4 to 6 weeks? Anything longer than that is too long. And lastly, please do not braid me back in with the extensions for at least 2 months.

Weave

I know you like trying out different styles and the weave was really cool. However, I didn't know how to tell you but it was really tight and heavy. In fact, the extra hair you added to me cut into me a little, so I was slightly worried about whether or not I would actually survive your last weave. I know you look really nice in it but honestly, I was suffering and was not sure whether I could take too much more.

Tight ponytails and buns

I think it is great being gathered up with my pals and put into a nice bun or ponytail, but again, does it have to be that tight? I felt like I was being permanently stretched and I wasn't sure this was going to be something I can deal with in the long term. I must ask you to loosen that style, please.

Traction Alopecia

If you feel pain while you are wearing any style, it is best to take it out because the chronic pulling of me into these styles can actually cause a type of hair loss, called *Traction Alopecia.* This is where I thin or I disappear from the edges of your scalp altogether. However, the good news is that if it is caught early enough, this condition can be reversed and I can regrow!

CHAPTER ELEVEN

DEPARTURE!

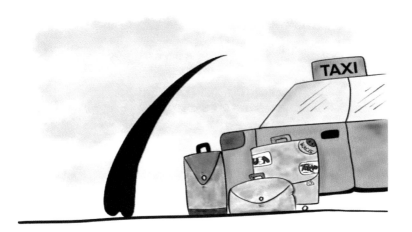

I have reached that final exit stage of the hair growth cycle, the Telogen Stage and I am actually getting ready to leave. I have had a good time and I am really pleased I survived it for so long on your scalp, despite the close shaves, so thanks for accommodating me. However, I would be grateful if you will - in the future - take the time and effort to look after the rest of my pals while I am away because I look forward to a bit of company when I return!

I will be taking a short break now, and if all goes well, I will be back!

Printed in Poland
by Amazon Fulfillment
Poland Sp. z o.o., Wrocław

51578688R00023